The Ultimate Guide To The Eat Clean Diet

It's a lifestyle choice

AMARPREET SINGH

Publisher - The Thought Flame

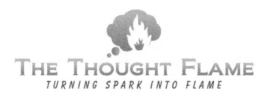

THE THOUGHT FLAME

TURNING SPARK INTO FLAME

info@thethoughtflame.com

www.thethoughtflame.com

Table of Contents

Introduction

The more progress that we make into the food industry and learn more about the kind of foods that we put into our systems, the more we better ourselves to eat healthier foods in the future.

Let's face it, most of the foods that we eat today are packed with harmful preservatives and unhealthy ingredients that, while they may taste delicious, will only harm us in the long run. Just because something tastes better does not necessarily mean that it is good for us.

However, over the years many people across the globe have taken it upon themselves to learn every aspect of the food industry and shed some light on the kind of harmful things that is being put into our food today. That is how the Eat Clean diet was born and how it has grown in popularity in the recent years.

In this eBook you will learn how the Eat Clean Diet came to be, the basics of this diet, what foods you can and cannot have and have a few recipes handy so that you can make them in the comfort of your own home.

So, what are you waiting for? Let's get started.

Chapter One: What Exactly Is The Eat Clean Diet?

If you have never heard of this diet before, I wouldn't be surprise. To answer this question I will give you the simplest answer possible. The Eat Clean diet is very straightforward and in all honesty shouldn't even count as a diet when it is more of a lifestyle. All the Eat Clean Diet entails is just a basic concept that revolves around the idea of what your food contains and where exactly it comes from. To simplify this answer even more, the whole point of this diet is to simply avoid eating any processed foods.

Processing foods means that food has already been processed once before. Some commonly processed foods consists of any kind of canned food, flour and many different types of food that has ingredients that you have never heard of before. There is no laws stating which foods are processed but they can range from anything from a simple hotdog to instant oatmeal.

So, what make processed foods really unhealthy? The main problem with these kinds of food is that after they have been processed most of the important nutrients that you need have been destroyed in the process. To make matters worse more additives are added to these already processed foods to help preserve the food just a tad longer and to improve its overall taste. These additives that are commonly added to food have been found to be linked to serious health problems such as cancer. If a type of food has the potential to cause cancer, why would you want it apart of your diet in the first place?

The Eat Clean Diet is all about the consumption of whole foods like fruits, vegetables, lean meats, healthy fats, and complex carbohydrates. The basic idea of Eat

Clean is not new. The principle behind this program has been rooted in the natural health movement since the 1960s. This health movement focused on the whole food approach to eating. It also promoted the consumption of unprocessed foods.

While the idea for this diet has been around for as long as anybody can remember, it wasn't widely known until Tosca Reno published a series of Eat Clean cookbooks. Reno is a Canadian fitness model that popularized this eating program and many people fell in love with it the moment he began talking about it. The principle is still the same as it was with the natural health movement in the 1960s, as foods are manufactured in the same way that they are today.

Who Is This Diet For?

The Eat Clean program is for people who want to make intelligent and healthier choices, that want to get fit, who want to feel better, and who want to limit their intake of processed food. Because this eating program is aimed towards the consumption of foods at their most natural and unprocessed form, taking part in it will enable your body to function at its best and, consequently, will make you feel fantastic and full of energy. This is far from the fad diets that have been lurking around, most of which make you feel lethargic, deprived, and hungry.

What This Diet Is Not?

If you're looking for another fad diet, then the Eat Clean program is not for you. The proponents of the program made it clear that this is not a diet but more of a way of life. If you're overweight, this program can help you lose those excess pounds. It can also help those who have problems in gaining weight.

Unlike other eating programs that you can find out there, it doesn't require you to starve yourself or make you count anything like calories, points, carbs, grams, and fat. You don't have to buy pre-packaged or pre-portioned food, and it doesn't require you to take pills or special potions. What this eating program calls for is the choice of choosing whole and natural foods.

You cannot get any healthier than participating in the Eat Clean lifestyle. When you rid yourself of consuming foods that will only serve to harm you, you will work towards creating a much healthier future for yourself.

Chapter Two: The Basics of The Eat Clean Diet and Everything That You Need To Know

If you have kept up on all of the latest trends in the health industry lately, then it is likely that you have heard about the Eat Clean Diet. Remember, the Eat Clean program is not a diet. This is a lifestyle choice as its proponents suggests. Unlike fad diets, eating clean won't promise that you'll lose any excess pounds. It doesn't even promote calorie or point counting. What it does instead is encourage healthy eating.

Before you can start following this program, it is important for you to get a handle on the basics of it first.

1. The Importance of Fruits and Veggies

Fruits and vegetables are important elements

of this eating program. While it is not the center of the Eat Clean program, the consumption of these foods is a basic part of it. Because fruits and vegetables are rich in vitamins and minerals, the American Cancer Society promotes the consumption of five servings of these foods a day.

Fruits and vegetables have cleansing and detoxifying properties. For instance, kale has detoxifying properties while celery eliminates excess fluids in the body. Apples also have healing compounds that get rid of carcinogenic toxins in the body. Lemons can eliminate putrefactive bacteria and mucous buildup in the intestines.

2. Eating Lean Protein Sources

Other than fruits and vegetables, the Eat Clean program also advocates a diet comprised of lean proteins. This includes plant-based proteins that are low in fat and high in fiber.

Examples of plant-based proteins include beans, legumes, tofu, and other soy-based products. Other sources of lean proteins include white meat poultry, fish, and lean cuts of beef.

Lean proteins are excellent sources of B vitamins, such as niacin and riboflavin, iron, magnesium, zinc, and vitamins E and C. B vitamins can help you raise your energy levels and improve nervous system function. Zinc, on the other hand, can help the immune system function normally.

3. Taking In Healthy Whole Grains

Because clean eating is all about eating foods in their most basic form, this includes the presence of whole grains. Whole grains are unprocessed foods that have a higher concentration of fiber and protein than their processed counterpart. Whole grains are good sources of energy but are low in saturated fat.

Whole grains are extremely popular in many dietary programs, and this is because it can help a dieter maintain weight and improve his health. According to studies, whole grains can help carotid arteries become healthier and reduce the risk of a variety of medical conditions such as colorectal cancer, heart problems, gum disease, and hypertension.

4. Drinking Plenty of Water

Other than healthy and natural food sources, another important part of eating clean is water. Sufficient intake of water is promoted by this eating and following this program. Unlike soda and other sugar-laden drinks, water has zero calories and doesn't contain any sugar. It helps regulate the body's functions and aids in improving one's metabolism. An intake of 8 glasses or more of water per day is advised.

Drinking the recommended amount of water per day can help you maintain the balance of fluids in your body. It can help maintain the right body temperature as well as improve circulation and transportation of nutrients.

5. Munch On A Few Healthy Snacks

If you plan on following this program you can forget about cookies, chips, and cakes. Eating Clean is not about those snacks since they are high in saturated fat. In this eating program, food options for snacks are still in line with the program's principle. Instead of pastries that are high in fat and drinks, which are overloaded with sugar, the Eat Clean program promotes healthy snacks such as fruits, nuts, vegetables, whole grain crackers, and low-fat milk or yogurt.

Don't be confused with what to and what not to eat. If you know the principle of eating clean by heart, then you don't have to fret over food choices. You'll know that to be healthy you just have to choose foods existing in their most natural form.

Chapter Three: The Benefits of Eating Clean and Common Mistakes To Avoid

Since the day that this diet was brought out into the light, the eat clean program has become a program that is extremely popular all across the world. However, its popularity did not come around simply because there was a large group of health-conscious people hanging around. Instead it grew in popularity thanks to people who were looking for new ways to change their eating habits into healthy ones.

Because of the success of this program, it is no secret how it gained such high acclaim from the general public and how it has managed to continue gaining followers even to this day. The benefits of eating clean have surpassed even those that have been claimed by different fad diets. In this chapter you will learn about the different benefits to following this program as well as common mistakes to avoid making to be as successful as you possibly can while following this program.

Health Benefits of Eating Clean

1. Improve Your Overall Energy Level

The most common source of body's energy is glucose. Glucose comes from the food you eat, particularly from carbohydrates. Carbohydrates are divided into two groups: complex and simple. In contrast to simple carbohydrates, complex carbohydrates make you feel full longer because they are composed of both starch and fiber. It takes some time for the body to process complex carbs.

Sources of complex carbohydrates such as whole grains, starchy vegetables, and legumes result to a sustained release of energy. By getting into the eating clean program, you will be able to improve your energy level and feel energized throughout the entire day. You will no longer be lethargic and will have sufficient energy to keep you going the entire day.

2. Get Enough Sleep Throughout The Night

The vitamins and minerals contained in the whole foods you consume in this diet can help regulate hormonal function. Healthy foods have calming effects on your nervous system and can help trigger a response of sleep-inducing hormone production. All of these can promote better sleep especially during night time. You are less likely to have difficulties sleeping at night and have insomnia.

3. Build A Stronger Immune System

Your overall health condition will improve once

you follow this program. The fruits, vegetables, yogurt and fermented food that you will consume can significantly help maintain a healthy number of probiotics in your digestive system. Probiotics can regulate your immune system response and make it healthy.

4. Have Healthier Skin and Hair

You don't have to spend too much money experimenting on products to fight acne, wrinkles, and look younger. This is because eating clean helps to promotes sufficient intake of water, which will help you achieve healthier looking skin. Aside from hydration, water flushes out toxins, giving you that natural glow.

Since you don't consume high-glycemic foods such as processed sugar in this diet, you will be less susceptible to acne and breakouts. The fruits and vegetables that you would be eating in this diet can also help you grow healthy hair. Consuming sufficient amounts of water can also hydrate, eliminate impurities and strengthen your hair.

5. Save Yourself A Bit of Money

Unlike fad diets, the eating clean program helps you to save more money. Processed and fast foods or those that are pre-packaged are not just unhealthy, but they will also cost you more than their homemade versions. Since you will become a much healthier person, you will be less prone to develop certain illnesses that require costly medications. This will save you from spending on treatments and surgical procedures that are needed to help you recover from ailments.

6. Reduce Your Risk of Getting Life Threatening Diseases

The risk for having lifestyle diseases such as hypertension, stroke, and diabetes will be greatly reduced with this eating clean program.

These diseases often stem from unhealthy foods such as those that contain sodium, fat, and sugar-laden food products, and practices such as sedentary lifestyle and smoking. With this program you will consume less artificial food additives, sugar, preservatives, and pesticides, which are the most popular causes of life-threatening conditions such as cancer.

Common Mistakes To Avoid Making While On This Program

When it comes to being successful with this program, it is best that you stick as tightly to the program as possible. Make sure that you follow every rule and principle religiously until it becomes second nature to you. Unfortunately, for many people who have tried this program before and failed often slack on the rules that they have to follow.

The good news is that you can avoid making a few simple mistakes when it comes to this program by paying close attention to certain guideline of the program and by making sure that you commit to learning about a few of these common Eating Clean mistakes that people tend to make.

Mistake #1: Choosing The Wrong Kind of Fat To Use

Because the Eat Clean diet is not a typical eating program, it promotes eating a well-balanced meal. This means a balanced combination of carbohydrates, lean meats, and fat is recommended. However, you should know that while fats are needed by the body for insulation, brain function, hormone health, and the like, indulging with this food group, especially the wrong kind, could turn your health back to its former, sorry state.

Not all fats are created the same. There are trans, saturated, and unsaturated fats. What you should include in your meal plans are foods that contain unsaturated fats. The two other fats, the trans and saturated fats, are responsible for the increasing incidence of lifestyle diseases, so limit your intake of them. Consume more unsaturated or healthy fats that can be found in olive oil, nuts, avocados and legumes.

Mistake #2: Missing Out On Breakfast

Skipping breakfast is another common mistake that you should avoid. Bear in mind that breakfast is the most important meal of the day. When you skip breakfast just because you're in a hurry, you'll end up hungry before lunch and eating sugary muffins or other unhealthy foods. You can have a vegetable smoothie for breakfast, as it will only take a few minutes to prepare the drink.

Mistake #3: Loading Up On Too Many Carbs

Just like fats, carbohydrates are also not created the same. It is sub-divided into two groups: the complex and simple carbohydrates. If you plan to start eating clean, then you should ditch your habit of loading up on too much starchy carbs. Compared to complex carbohydrates, starchy or simple carbohydrates don't contain as much as fiber and nutrients as unprocessed ones. Because starchy carbs often lead to a sudden surge and crash of your glucose level, you end up snacking all throughout the day. As mentioned in the previous chapter, it is best that you pair starchy carbs with lean protein to stabilize your insulin levels.

Mistake #4: Not Eating Enough

Not eating enough food won't make you slimmer and healthier. Although it is true that you won't ingest calories while starving yourself, the effects are only temporary. If you continue to deprive your body with the amount of nutrients it needs, your metabolism will slow down. This will stop your body from burning energy and encourage it to store more fat. In other words, you will become very tired, oversleep, and weak. Make sure that you eat according to how this diet should be practiced.

These are the most common mistakes of people following the Eat Clean program. Many people think that just because the food is low in calories, it's also healthy, which isn't necessarily true.

By learning about the common mistakes that people tend to make while following this program, you can help ensure that you will not make the same and give yourself a chance to be more successful with the program in the long run. Whether you are on this program in the first place to live a healthier lifestyle or whether you are looking for a way to ensure that you eat on the healthiest of food, you simply cannot go wrong with the Eat Clean program.

Chapter Four: My Recommended Grocery List

If you are new to this program, there is a chance that you are clueless about what you should stock your home with in terms of food. I mean, there are several food items out there today that are packed with the very thing that you are trying to avoid.

Well, not you don't need to worry. This chapter is solely dedicated to helping you stock your home with the healthiest foods possible while also helping you to transition into this program comfortably. Change up the list accordingly depending on your specific tastes and don't worry if you miss getting an item or two. You always have time to get it later.

Fresh Veggies/Herbs

- Plenty of Lettuce

- Tomatoes
- Kale
- Parsley
- Potatoes
- Onions
- Plenty of Garlic
- Cilantro
- Broccoli

Fresh Fruits

- Plenty of Avocados
- Mixed Berries
- Apples
- Grapes (Green or Purple)
- Bananas
- Melon

Drinks

- Milk, Almond or Hemp Preferable
- Teas, Plenty of Herbal Ones

- Coconut Water

Protein and Grain Sources

- Black Beans
- Flaxseed
- Brown Rice
- Lentils
- Almonds, Raw
- Almond Butter
- Cannellini Beans
- Millet
- Chickpeas
- Cashews, Raw
- Pinto Beans
- Sunflower Seeds
- Walnuts

Healthy Snacks

- Popcorn
- Soups, Organic and Canned

- Cheese Shreds, Dairy-Free
- Tortilla Chips
- Chocolate, Raw
- Frozen Fruit Smoothies
- Frozen Veggies
- Pretzels

Condiments To Use For Flavoring

- Coconut Oil
- Maple Syrup
- Olive Oil, Extra Virgin
- Hot Sauce, Your Favorite Brand
- Cinnamon, Ground
- Black Pepper
- Sesame Oil
- Red Pepper Flakes
- Cayenne Pepper, Ground
- Turmeric, Ground

A Few Things To Keep In Mind...

When it comes to getting together you shopping list, make sure that you pick out the freshest foods possible. You'll be able to tell immediately which foods are fresh and which are not and before you know it you will be able to tell the difference immediately.

Also be aware of what items you buy that may be processed. There are certain food items and cooking ingredients that are processed but are not marketed as such. There are also grocery items that are minimally processed such as those cooked at high temperature for too long. There are also items that are extensively processed such as those with many ingredients. Exercise care in choosing the items that you put in your cart. Always remember that it can be difficult to find items that have not went through processing or treatments.

Chapter Five: A Few Easy and Delicious Eat Clean Program Recipes

Now that you know how the eat clean program can help to benefit you, know exactly what mistakes to avoid in the future and what the entire point of this program is, it is time to begin preparing your healthy eat clean meals.

Each recipe that you will find in this eBook follows the guidelines to the eat clean program religiously and each recipe that you find is incredibly delicious, allowing you to enjoy your meals with the peace of mind that you are not putting anything potentially harmful into your system.

So, what are you waiting for? Let's get cooking!

Eat Clean Appetizer Recipes

Bruschetta Alla Guacamole

Avocado is a source of good fat and is considered to be one of the most versatile fruits out there. With this recipe you will have the perfect combination that will help yield a rich and delicious tasting bruschetta, making it a perfect dish to make as an appetizer.

Total Cook Time: 25 Minutes

Makes: 8 Servings

Ingredients:

8 Slices of Bread, Whole Grain

1 Avocado, Ripe

2 Cloves of Garlic, Minced

1 Tomato, Ripe and Diced Finely

1 Cucumber, Fresh and Diced Finely

1 Onion, Green and Chopped Finely

1 Tbsp. of Lemon Juice

1 Tbsp. of Cilantro, Chopped Finely

Dash of Salt and Pepper For Taste

Directions:

1. Take your whole grain bread and toast it to your desired color. Place the toasted bread onto a platter.

2. Next mash up your avocado in a small sized mixing bowl. Then stir in your tomato, lemon juice, garlic, onion and cilantro. Stir thoroughly until evenly combined.

3. Season with your dash of salt and pepper and spoon your mixture right on top of your toasted bread slice. Serve immediately and enjoy.

Fresh Mozzarella and Tomato Skewers

This is one of the fastest appetizer recipes that you will ever make. They look beautiful and are packed full of fresh taste, giving you a dish that you won't soon forget. While it may be a simple recipe to make, this is a dish that will certainly shine at your dinner table.

Total Cook Time: 20 Minutes

Makes: 6 Servings

Ingredients:

2 Cups of Tomatoes, Cherry and Fresh

6 Ounces of Mozzarella, Fresh and Cut Into Small Cubes or Balls

6 Leaves of Basil, Fresh

Dash of Salt and Pepper For Taste

2 Tbsp. of Olive Oil

A Handful of Skewers or Toothpicks, Wooden

Directions:

1. Gently place your fresh mozzarella and tomatoes onto your wooden skewers or toothpicks.

2. Then garnish your skewers with your basil leaves and dash of salt and pepper. Place them onto a serving plate and drizzle with a touch of olive oil. Serve immediately and enjoy.

Cucumber and Cream Cheese Cups

This is a great idea for a recipe especially if you are looking to serve a fresh appetizer that is incredibly low in calories. The filling that you will use in this recipe is low in fat and tastes great, allowing you to enjoy this dish without having to feel guilty about it.

Total Cook Time: 30 Minutes

Makes: 4 Servings

Ingredients:

2 Cucumbers, Fresh and Sliced Into Thick Slices

½ Cup of Cream Cheese, Low In Fat and Softened

1 Clove of Garlic, Minced

1 Tbsp. of Dill, Finely Chopped

1 Tbsp. of Parsley, Finely Chopped

Dash of Salt and Pepper For Taste

Directions:

1. Slice up your fresh cucumber and scoop out

some of the flesh of the cucumber to help form your "cups." Place the "cups" onto a serving dish.

2. In a small sized mixing bowl mix together your parsley, cream cheese, dill and garlic together until evenly mixed. Next add your dash of salt and pepper for taste and spoon the mixture into your "cups."

3. Serve while still fresh and enjoy immediately.

Miniature Spinach Pizzas

It is no secret that spinach is one of the healthiest vegetables that you can have today. However, it is hard to include in everyone's diet simply because to many people it does not taste good. With this recipe you do not have to worry about that because who doesn't love a great tasting pizza?

Total Cook Time: 30 Minutes

Makes: 6 Servings

Ingredients:

6 Pita Breads, Whole Wheat

½ Cup of Tomato Sauce, Fresh or Canned

1 Cup of Spinach Leaves, Fresh and Left Whole

1 Cup of Mozzarella Cheese, Fresh and Shredded

Dash of Salt and Pepper For Taste

Directions:

1. Preheat your oven to 350 degrees. While your oven heats up place your whole grain pita bread onto a baking sheet.

2. Brush each pita bread slice with your fresh tomato sauce and cover with a layer of fresh spinach and shredded mozzarella cheese. Season with your dash of salt and pepper.

3. Place your baking sheet into your oven and allow to bake for the next 10 to 15 minutes or until the mozzarella has fully melted and the tops are crusty.

4. Remove from oven and either serve immediately or serve once completely chilled. Enjoy.

Delicious Eat Clean Soup Recipes

Savory Cauliflower and Garlic Soup

While cauliflower is relatively mild in flavor, it can take a lot of seasoning in order to make it taste better. No better seasoning helps than garlic and some black pepper. This soup is an extremely creamy and savory soup, which will surely please even the pickiest of eaters.

Total Cook Time: 45 Minutes

Makes: 6 Servings

Ingredients:

2 Tbsp. of Olive Oil

1 Onion, Medium In Size and Finely Chopped

4 Cloves of Garlic, Finely Chopped

1 Head of Cauliflower, Fresh and Sliced Into Florets

4 Cups of Vegetable Stock, Low In Sodium

Dash of Salt and Pepper For Taste

½ of a Lemon, Fresh and Juiced

¼ tsp. of Cumin Powder, Ground

Directions:

1. Using a large sized soup pot, heat up your olive oil and add in your minced garlic and chopped onion. Sauté them both for the next 2 minutes or until fragrant.

2. Next add in your cauliflower and vegetable stock. Season with your dash of salt and pepper. On medium heat allow your soup to cook for the next 20 minutes.

3. After 20 minutes add in your cumin powder

and fresh lemon juice. Remove from heat and transfer soup into a blender. Puree your soup until it reaches the desired consistency.

4. Pour into a few serving bowls and serve while still warm. Enjoy.

Thai Style Tomato Soup

While this tomato soup looks anything but different when you first look at it, but the moment that you taste it for the first time you will immediately taste all of those wonderful Thai flavors that will send your taste buds straight to heaven. There is no need to add anything more to this dish as it already has everything you are looking for.

Total Cook Time: 45 Minutes

Makes: 6 Servings

Ingredients:

2 Tbsp. of Olive Oil

1 Shallot, Medium In Size and Chopped Finely

2 Cloves of Garlic, Finely Chopped

12 Inches of Grass Stalk, Lemon and Crushed

4 Tomatoes, Heirloom, Peeled and Chopped Finely

1 tsp. of Ginger, Grated

Dash of Salt and Pepper

3 Cups of Vegetable Stock

1 tsp. of Hot Sauce, Your Favorite Brand

Directions:

1. Using a large sized soup pot, heat up your olive oil over medium to high heat and then add in your minced garlic and chopped shallot. Sauté these for the next 2 minutes or until fragrant.

2. Then add in the rest of your ingredients and allow the soup to cook for the next 20 to 25 minutes.

3. Remove from heat and toss out your lemongrass stalk. Pour your soup into a blender and puree your soup until it reaches the desired consistency that you want.

4. Pour your soup into serving bowls and serve either warm or chilled. Enjoy.

Healthy Cabbage Soup

This recipe takes ordinary cabbage and turns it into a completely delicious and filling soup that will leave you wanting more. This soup recipe is incredibly light and healthy, making it one of the healthiest soup recipes that you will find.

Total Cook Time: 45 Minutes

Makes: 8 Servings

Ingredients:

2 Tbsp. of Olive Oil

1 Red Bell Pepper, Cored and Sliced Finely

1 Green Bell Pepper, Cored and Sliced Finely

1 Onion, Medium In Size and Chopped Finely

3 Cups of Water, Warm

1 Head of Cabbage, Shredded

2 Tbsp. of Tomato Paste, Fresh

½ Of A Lemon, Juiced

Dash of Salt and Pepper For Taste

1 Tbsp. of Cilantro, Chopped Finely

1 tsp. of Thyme, Dried

Directions:

1. Using a large sized saucepan, heat up your olive oil over medium to high heat. Add in your onion and sauté it for the next 2 to 3 minutes.

2. Next add in your peppers and cabbage and allow to cook for the next 5 minutes. After 5 minutes add in your water and tomato paste. Stir until combined evenly. Then add in your dash of salt and pepper for taste and stir again.

3. Allow the soup to cook over medium heat for the next 20 to 30 minutes. After this time add in the rest of your ingredients and stir to combine evenly.

4. Serve into bowls and enjoy immediately.

Fall Seasoned Soup

This soup is the perfect combination of what you love about fall: colorful bell peppers, savory squash and ripe tomatoes. Once pureed the ingredients used in this soup recipe will give it a creamy and rich texture, making it a dish that you are going to want to make during the fall months.

Total Cook Time: 45 Minutes

Makes: 8 Servings

Ingredients:

2 Tbsp. of Olive Oil

1 Clove of Garlic, Chopped Finely

1 Onion, Medium In Size and Finely Chopped

4 Cups of Butternut Squash, Chopped Into Cubes

1 Pinch of Cinnamon Powder, Ground

1 Pinch of Cardamom, Ground

1 Tomato, Ripe and Finely Chopped

3 Cups of Vegetable Stock, Low In Sodium

¼ tsp. of Anise Seeds

1 Red Bell Pepper, Cored and Chopped Finely

1 Cup of Water, Warm

Dash of Salt and Pepper For Taste

¼ Cup of Walnuts, Chopped and To Be Used For Serving

Directions:

1. Using a large soup pot, heat up your olive oil over medium heat. Add in your onion and garlic and sauté for the next 2 minutes or until fragrant.

2. Then stir in the rest of your ingredients except for the chopped walnuts until evenly combined. Allow to cook for the next 20 to 30 minutes.

3. Remove from heat and pour into a blender to puree until it reaches the right consistency. Serve and top with chopped walnuts. Enjoy.

Filling Eat Clean Salad Recipes

Traditional Mexican Bean Salad

This delicious salad is made up of delicious avocado, corn and beans, making it possibly the richest salad you will ever taste. Since it is Mexican, it wouldn't be fitting if there wasn't a touch of spice thrown in there.

Total Cook Time: 20 Minutes

Makes: 6 Servings

Ingredients:

1 Small Can of Black Beans, Drained and Rinsed

1 Small Can of Corn, Sweet, Drained and Rinsed

1 Cucumber, Fresh and Sliced Thinly

½ Cup of Cilantro, Finely Chopped

1 Tomato, Ripe, Fresh and Cut Into Small Cubes

1 Avocado, Ripe, Peeled and Sliced Finely

2 Tbsp. of Olive Oil

2 Limes, Fresh and Juiced

Dash of Salt and Pepper For Taste

½ tsp. of Oregano, Dried

Directions:

1. In a small sized mixing bowl, combine all of your ingredients together and toss softly until thoroughly combined.

2. Serve once thoroughly tossed and enjoy.

Fresh Spinach and Strawberry Salad

If you are looking for a salad that will send your taste buds into heaven, this is the salad recipe for you. Mixed with a bomb of tasty flavors, you will be able to enjoy a highly nutritious and delicious dish.

Total Cook Time: 20 Minutes

Makes: 4 Servings

Ingredients:

1 Pound of Spinach, Baby and Shredded

½ Cup of Strawberries, Pureed Finely

1 Cup of Strawberries, Sliced Into Halves

2 Tbsp. of Olive Oil

½ Of A Lemon, Juiced

Dash of Salt and Pepper For Taste

1 tsp. of Vinegar, Balsamic

1 tsp. of Honey

Directions:

1. Place your fresh spinach onto a serving plate then place your freshly cut strawberries on top of that and set aside.

2. To make the dressing you will need to combine the rest on your ingredients in a small bowl until combined thoroughly.

3. Drizzle your dressing over your salad and serve immediately. Enjoy.

Grilled Balsamic Veggie Salad

If you are looking for a salad recipe that will enhance the natural flavor and sweetness of your veggies, this is the salad recipe for you. While still preserving all of the important nutrients this recipe will bring you a dish that tastes smoky and is absolutely delicious.

Total Cook Time: 35 Minutes

Makes: 6 Servings

Ingredients:

1 Zucchini, Fresh and Sliced Thinly

1 Eggplant, Fresh, Peeled and Sliced Thinly

2 Tomatoes, Ripe and Sliced Finely

1 Carrot, Fresh and Cut Lengthwise Very Finely

1 Onion, Red In Color and Sliced Finely

2 Yellow Bell Pepper, Fresh, Cored and Sliced Into Quarters

2 Tbsp. of Olive Oil

¼ Cup of Vinegar, Balsamic

Dash of Salt and Pepper For Taste

4 Cloves of Garlic, Chopped Finely

Directions:

1. Using a medium sized saucepan, heat it over high heat and place all of your vegetables into it, one by one.

2. Sauté your veggies until they are brown on each side and then remove from heat. Place them into a medium sized mixing bowl.

3. Using a separate bowl mix up your balsamic vinegar, dash of salt and pepper for taste, olive oil and garlic together until evenly combined.

4. Pour your new dressing over your grilled veggies and serve immediately. Enjoy.

Avocado and Spinach Salad

The best part about this salad can be either the rich flavor of the poppy seeds that you use for the dressing or the creamy texture of the avocado. The contrast between these two ingredients help make this a dish that is both filling and delicious.

Total Cook Time: 20 Minutes

Makes: 6 Servings

Ingredients:

2 Tbsp. of Almonds, Sliced

1 Pound of Spinach, Baby

1 Avocado, Ripe, peeled and Sliced

1 Tbsp. of Poppy Seeds

½ of A Lemon, juiced

1 tsp. of Honey

1 tsp. of Lemon Zest, Fresh

1 Tbsp. of Olive Oil

Dash of Salt and Pepper For Taste

1 tsp. of Vinegar, Apple Cider

Directions:

1. In a salad bowl combine your avocado, spinach and almonds until gently mixed together.

2. In a small sized mixing bowl combine the rest of your ingredients together to make your dressing. Stir together until thoroughly mixed.

3. Drizzle your dressing over your salad and serve while as fresh as possible.

Conclusion

In this fast moving world of ours, one of the things that we tend to neglect the most is our overall health. Almost every person on the planet is too busy chasing their dreams or stressing themselves out over their careers when their overall health should be the first thing that they should be worrying about.

Because of this it is no longer a surprise as to why so many people choose to settle for foods that are quick to make and that are fully processed rather than enjoy a home cooked and healthy meal right from the comfort of their own home. The sad part about this is, while yes, these foods may simply be easier on us all around; we will pay for it eventually.

With the many illnesses and diseases that we can get nowadays should be proof enough why changing what we eat is ultimately important if we wish to live longer and healthier lives.

While this program may be far from perfect and while it is not free from criticism, the Eat Clean program is certainly one of the healthiest out there today. However, the choice to live a healthier life and to eat foods that are not processed is completely up to you. You are the only one who is control of your body and you life, and if you want to live a healthier lifestyle, changing to the Eat Clean diet is one that only you can make for yourself.

About Us

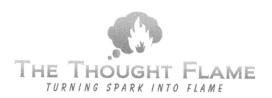

The Thought Flame is committed to add value to its customers through various books, online courses and other resources. You can learn more about us and our books at www.thethoughtflame.com.

Don't forget to check out our amazing **online video courses** at www.thethoughtflame.com/courses/ to take your knowledge to another level.

To check out our **extraordinary collection of diet/cookbooks**, visit http://www.thethoughtflame.com/category/non-fictional/cookbooks/ .

As a part of our valued relationship with our customers, we keep providing you free promotional books, courses and other stuff on subscribing with us on our site. We have a strict anti-spam policy and assure you no spam mails will be sent to your mailbox.

To subscribe with us, visit www.thethoughtflame.com.

Like our work and would like to say thanks?

Buy us a cup of coffee at www.thethoughtflame.com/coffee/

Author

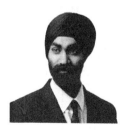

Amarpreet Singh is an avid learner and his passion for education has made him travel, work and study all across the world. He holds three masters degrees, including MBA, from top universities in Asia.

He is author of dozens of books, many of which are Amazon's bestseller, varying in various topics and categories. He also teaches many online courses having thousands of students across the world.

He has a keen interest in international affairs, economics, global poverty and politics, financial markets and entrepreneurship, and strives to be part of a community that shares the same passion.

He has worked as consultant with organizations like Airbus and The World Bank.

He loves travelling and learning about new cultures, and has been fortunate to live/work/travel/study in countries like India, China, Korea, US, South Africa, Japan, Philippines, Singapore, Canada etc., and learn about the culture and lifestyle in each of them.

To check out more of his work, visit

www.thethoughtflame.com

Made in United States
Orlando, FL
20 November 2024

54181320R00039